Common Drugs in Canadian Care

A Nurse's Drug Guide to Hospitals and Long-Term Facilities

M.A. Gorre

DISCLAIMER

The information contained in this book is intended for educational and informational purposes only. It is not a substitute for professional medical advice, diagnosis, or treatment. While every effort has been made to ensure the accuracy of the content, the author, publishers, and distributors cannot be held responsible for the validity of the information presented or for the outcomes resulting from the application of this information.

Healthcare professionals should exercise their own clinical judgment when interpreting the information and applying it to patient care. The medications and treatments discussed in this book are subject to change as medical research and practice continue to evolve. Always consult with qualified healthcare providers for diagnosis and treatment, and for the most current and comprehensive medical information relevant to your specific needs.

The author and publishers disclaim all responsibility for any liability, loss, or risk, personal or otherwise, which is incurred as a consequence, directly or indirectly, of the use and application of any of the contents of this book.

Contents

Introduction

Hello and welcome to this comprehensive guide on common medications used in long-term care facilities and Hospitals. I've been a dedicated nurse for nearly 15 years. During this time, I've been privileged to work in diverse settings, ranging from emergency rooms to geriatric wards, where I've encountered a broad spectrum of medications and their applications.

Medication use in healthcare settings is both a science and an art. While medical science provides us with the basis for understanding the effects and appropriate use of medications, the art lies in the individualized care that each patient requires. Correct medication administration is critical, as it directly influences patient outcomes and the overall quality of healthcare services.

I've written this book to serve as a practical resource for my fellow healthcare providers, particularly nurses who are the backbone of medication administration in medical settings. However, this guide is also designed for anyone interested in understanding common medications' basics, uses, risks, and benefits.

In this book, you will find a detailed yet easily understandable outline for each medication, featuring its generic name, market brand names, classification, and much more. For ease of use, I've also included whether the drug is available Over-The-Counter (OTC), its mechanism of action explained in layperson's terms, indications, contraindications, typical side effects, and nursing considerations. Plus, each entry follows a standardized format, ensuring that the information you need is where you expect it to be.

In pursuing excellent patient care, it's vital to continually educate ourselves and keep our knowledge up-to-date. Whether you're an experienced healthcare provider or someone newly qualified, I hope this book serves as an invaluable reference guide in your daily work and contributes to improving patient care.

Thank you for picking up this guide, and I wish you all the best in your professional journey.

Warm regards,
M.A. GORRE

Proper Administration of Oral Medications

Twelve Rights of Medication Administration

1. **Right Patient**: Confirm the patient's identity using at least two identifiers, like name and date of birth.

2. **Right Medication and Expiration**: Double-check the medication against the prescription. Make sure it has not expired.

3. **Right Dose**: Measure the prescribed dose carefully, using the appropriate instrument.

4. **Right Route**: Confirm that the medication should be given via the intended route (oral, IV, etc.).

5. **Right Time**: Administer the medication at the time prescribed.

6. **Right Documentation**: Record all pertinent information, including medication, dose, time, and any patient reactions.

7. **Right Reason**: Understand the reason for the medication and educate the patient as necessary.

8. **Right to Refuse**: Acknowledge that the patient has the right to refuse medication; their decision should be respected and documented.

9. **Right Response**: Monitor the patient for the expected effects and any possible side effects.

10. **Right Education**: Provide necessary education to the patient or caregiver about the medication.

11. **Right Evaluation**: After administration, evaluate the patient's response to the medication, both therapeutically and for any adverse reactions.

12. **Right to Know**: Ensure the patient and their caregivers understand what medication is being administered, why it is being administered, and what the potential side effects may be.

Important Tips for Administering Oral Medications

1. **Preparation**: Make sure to wash your hands and prepare a clean area before handling medications.

2. **Gloves**: Use gloves when handling medication, especially if the medication is toxic or can be absorbed through the skin.

3. **No Crushing**: Do not crush or break tablets or capsules unless approved by a healthcare provider.

4. **Liquid Medications**: Use a calibrated dropper or cup to measure liquid medications.

5. **Water**: Administer oral medications with a full glass of water, unless contraindicated.

6. **Food**: Follow any food restrictions; some medications should be taken with food, while others should be taken on an empty stomach.

7. **Patient Position**: Make sure the patient is in an appropriate position for swallowing, usually sitting up or slightly reclined.

8. **Check Expiration Dates**: Always check the expiration date on the medication bottle or packaging.

9. **Double-Check**: Verify for allergies and potential interactions with other medications the patient is taking.

10. **Storage**: Store medications according to manufacturer's guidelines.

11. **Disposal**: Dispose of expired medications properly, following facility guidelines or manufacturer instructions.

ACETAMINOPHEN

Brand Names: Tylenol, Panadol

OTC Availability: Yes

Classification: Analgesic, Antipyretic

Mechanism of Action: Inhibits COX enzymes, leading to reduced pain and fever. The exact mechanism is not fully understood.

Indications:

- Mild to moderate pain

- Fever

Contraindications:

- Severe liver disease

- Hypersensitivity to acetaminophen

Side Effects:

- Liver toxicity at high doses

- Nausea

- Rash

Nursing Considerations:

- Assess level of pain and/or fever.

- Monitor liver function in prolonged use or if patient has history of liver disease.

Administration: Can be taken with or without food. Taking it with food may minimize stomach upset.

Additional Information:

- Risk of liver toxicity increases with alcohol consumption.

- Available in various forms such as oral, rectal, and intravenous.

ALBUTEROL

Brand Names: Ventolin, Proventil

OTC Availability: No

Classification: Short-Acting Beta-2 Agonist

Mechanism of Action: Stimulates beta-2 receptors in the lungs, causing bronchial smooth muscle relaxation.

Indications:

- Asthma

- Chronic Obstructive Pulmonary Disease (COPD)

Contraindications:

- Hypersensitivity to albuterol

- Cardiac arrhythmias associated with tachycardia

Side Effects:

- Tremors

- Palpitations

- Nervousness

- Hypokalemia

Nursing Considerations:

- Assess respiratory status before and after use.

- Monitor heart rate.

- Educate on proper inhaler technique.

- Inform patients to avoid overuse and to report worsening symptoms.

Additional Information:

- Available in various forms including inhalers and nebulizer solutions.

- Rapid onset but short duration; not intended for long-term control.

- Interacts with some medications like beta-blockers.

AMOXICILLIN

Brand Names: Amoxil, Moxatag

OTC Availability: No

Classification: Antibiotic (Penicillin Class)

Mechanism of Action: Inhibits bacterial cell wall synthesis, leading to cell death.

Indications:

- Bacterial infections like strep throat, ear infections, pneumonia

- Urinary tract infections

- Dental abscesses

Contraindications:

- Hypersensitivity to penicillin or other beta-lactam antibiotics

- History of severe allergic reaction to antibiotics

Side Effects:
- Diarrhea

- Nausea

- Rash

- Vomiting

- Yeast infections

Nursing Considerations:
- Assess infection symptoms before and during treatment.

- Monitor for allergic reactions.

- Educate patients on completing the full antibiotic course even if they feel better.

- Advise patients to report severe diarrhea or other adverse effects.

- Monitor renal and hepatic function in long-term use.

Additional Information:
- Available in various forms including capsules, chewable tablets, and liquids.

- Should be taken with food to improve absorption.

- Interaction with other medications like oral contraceptives may reduce efficacy.

AMLODIPINE

Brand Names: Norvasc

OTC Availability: No

Classification: Calcium Channel Blocker

Mechanism of Action: Inhibits calcium ions from entering vascular smooth muscle cells, leading to vasodilation.

Indications:

- Hypertension

- Angina

Contraindications:

- Severe hypotension

- Aortic stenosis

- Hypersensitivity to amlodipine

Side Effects:
- Dizziness

- Swelling of the lower extremities

- Flushing

- Palpitations

Nursing Considerations:
- Monitor blood pressure and heart rate regularly.

- Assess for symptoms of angina.

- Educate patients on orthostatic precautions due to risk of dizziness.

- Instruct patients to report side effects like severe swelling or prolonged hypotension.

Additional Information:
- Dose adjustment may be needed in liver impairment.

- May interact with medications like simvastatin, increasing risk of side effects.

ASPIRIN

Brand Names: Bayer, Ascriptin, Bufferin

OTC Availability: Yes

Classification: Nonsteroidal Anti-Inflammatory Drug (NSAID), Antiplatelet

Mechanism of Action: Inhibits COX enzymes, reducing the production of prostaglandins and thromboxanes, thereby reducing inflammation, pain, and blood clotting.

Indications:

- Mild to moderate pain (e.g., headache, toothache)

- Inflammation (e.g., arthritis)

- Fever reduction

- Prevention of heart attacks and strokes

Contraindications:

- Peptic ulcer disease

- Hemorrhagic stroke

- Severe renal or hepatic impairment

- Hypersensitivity to aspirin or other NSAIDs

- Children and teenagers with viral infections due to the risk of Reye's syndrome

Side Effects:

- Gastrointestinal bleeding or ulcers

- Tinnitus (ringing in the ears)

- Increased bleeding time

- Nausea or vomiting

Nursing Considerations:

- Assess pain and temperature before administration.

- Monitor for signs of gastrointestinal bleeding.

- Be cautious in patients with a history of ulcers, kidney disease, or those taking anticoagulant medications.

- Instruct patients to take with food or milk to minimize gastric irritation.

- Monitor platelet count and liver and kidney function tests during long-term use.

Additional Information:

- Aspirin is commonly used in low doses as an antiplatelet agent to prevent heart attacks and strokes; confirm the indication for use.

- Inform patients about the risk of increased bleeding, especially before surgeries or dental procedures.

- Encourage patients to report any unusual symptoms such as severe abdominal pain, black or tarry stools, or any unusual bleeding.

- Aspirin should not be given to children or teenagers with fever due to the risk of Reye's syndrome, a rare but serious condition.

ATENOLOL

Brand Names: Tenormin

OTC Availability: No

Classification: Beta-Blocker

Mechanism of Action: Blocks beta-1 adrenergic receptors, reducing heart rate and blood pressure.

Indications:

- Hypertension

- Angina

- Cardiac arrhythmias

Contraindications:

- Heart block

- Severe bradycardia

- Decompensated heart failure

Side Effects:
- Fatigue

- Dizziness

- Bradycardia

- Cold hands and feet

Nursing Considerations:
- Monitor blood pressure and heart rate.

- Assess for symptoms of heart failure.

- Caution in patients with asthma or respiratory conditions.

- Educate on orthostatic precautions.

Additional Information:
- Abrupt withdrawal may worsen angina or precipitate arrhythmias.

- Use caution when combining with other medications that lower heart rate.

- Not the first choice for hypertension in some guidelines due to less protection for strokes.

ATORVASTATIN

Brand Names: Lipitor

OTC Availability: No

Classification: HMG-CoA Reductase Inhibitor (Statins)

Mechanism of Action: Inhibits the enzyme responsible for cholesterol synthesis in the liver.

Indications:

- Hyperlipidemia

- Prevention of cardiovascular events

Contraindications:

- Liver disease

- Pregnancy and lactation

- Hypersensitivity to atorvastatin

Side Effects:

- Muscle pain

- Liver dysfunction

- Gastrointestinal symptoms (nausea, diarrhea)

- Increased blood sugar levels

Nursing Considerations:

- Monitor lipid profile regularly.

- Assess for history of liver disease or high alcohol intake.

- Educate patients about lifestyle changes alongside medication.

- Monitor for muscle pain and liver function tests.

- Inform patients to avoid grapefruit juice due to interaction.

Additional Information:

- Dose often adjusted based on lipid levels.

- Caution is advised in patients also taking other medications affecting the liver.

- Long-term therapy may require regular ophthalmic exams.

AZITHROMYCIN

Brand Names: Zithromax, Z-Pak

OTC Availability: No

Classification: Antibiotic (Macrolide Class)

Mechanism of Action: Inhibits protein synthesis in bacteria, leading to cell death.

Indications:

- Respiratory tract infections

- Skin infections

- Sexually transmitted diseases like chlamydia

Contraindications:

- Liver disease

- Hypersensitivity to azithromycin or other macrolide antibiotics

- Heart arrhythmias

Side Effects:
- Diarrhea

- Nausea

- Abdominal pain

- Vomiting

Nursing Considerations:
- Assess infection symptoms before and during treatment.

- Monitor for allergic reactions.

- Educate patients on completing the full antibiotic course even if they feel better.

- Monitor liver and kidney function tests.

- Be cautious in patients with QT prolongation or other cardiac issues.

Additional Information:
- Often preferred for its shorter treatment course compared to other antibiotics.

- May interact with other medications like antacids, affecting absorption.

- Caution in patients with pre-existing liver conditions.

BISACODYL

Brand Names: Dulcolax, Fleet

OTC Availability: Yes

Classification: Stimulant Laxative

Mechanism of Action: Increases peristalsis by irritating the smooth muscle of the intestines.

Indications:

- Constipation

Contraindications:

- Bowel obstruction

- Acute abdominal conditions

Side Effects:

- Abdominal cramps

- Nausea

- Diarrhea

Nursing Considerations:

- Assess bowel function.

- Not for long-term use.

Administration: Oral or rectal; if oral, take with a full glass of water and avoid antacids or milk.

BUPROPION

Brand Names: Wellbutrin, Zyban

OTC Availability: No

Classification: Antidepressant (Atypical)

Mechanism of Action: Inhibits the reuptake of dopamine and norepinephrine.

Indications:

- Depression

- Smoking cessation

Contraindications:

- Seizure disorders

- History of eating disorders

- Concurrent use of MAOIs

Side Effects:

- Insomnia

- Dry mouth

- Increased heart rate

- Nausea

Nursing Considerations:

- Assess mental status and mood.

- Monitor for suicidal ideation, especially in adolescents.

- Educate on the risk of seizures and other side effects.

- Instruct patients not to stop medication abruptly.

Additional Information:

- Available in various formulations including SR and XL for extended release.

- Should not be used in conjunction with other medications that lower seizure threshold.

- Alcohol may interact with this medication.

CEFUROXIME

Brand Names: Ceftin, Zinacef

OTC Availability: No

Classification: Second-Generation Cephalosporin Antibiotic

Mechanism of Action: Inhibits bacterial cell wall synthesis.

Indications:

- Respiratory tract infections

- Urinary tract infections

- Skin and soft tissue infections

Contraindications:

- Hypersensitivity to cephalosporins or related antibiotics

Side Effects:

- Diarrhea

- Nausea

- Vomiting

Nursing Considerations:

- Monitor for signs of an allergic reaction.

- Assess renal and liver function.

Administration: Take with food to enhance absorption.

Additional Information:

- Complete the full course of treatment even if symptoms improve.

- Be cautious in patients with a history of penicillin allergy as cross-reactivity may occur.

CEPHALEXIN

Brand Names: Keflex, Biocef

OTC Availability: No

Classification: First-Generation Cephalosporin Antibiotic

Mechanism of Action: Inhibits bacterial cell wall synthesis.

Indications:

- Skin and soft tissue infections

- Urinary tract infections

- Respiratory tract infections

Contraindications:

- Hypersensitivity to cephalosporins or related antibiotics

Side Effects:

- Diarrhea

- Nausea

- Allergic reactions

Nursing Considerations:

- Monitor for signs of an allergic reaction.

- Assess renal function if indicated.

Administration: Can be taken with or without food; if gastrointestinal upset occurs, take with food.

Additional Information:

- Complete full course of treatment even if symptoms improve.

- Be cautious in patients with a history of penicillin allergy as cross-reactivity may occur.

CELECOXIB

Brand Names: Celebrex

OTC Availability: No

Classification: Nonsteroidal Anti-Inflammatory Drug (COX-2 inhibitor)

Mechanism of Action: Selectively inhibits COX-2 enzyme, reducing inflammation and pain.

Indications:

- Osteoarthritis

- Rheumatoid arthritis

- Acute pain

Contraindications:

- Hypersensitivity to celecoxib or sulfonamides

- History of cardiovascular or gastrointestinal bleeding

- Severe hepatic impairment

Side Effects:

- Gastrointestinal bleeding

- Hypertension

- Kidney dysfunction

- Allergic reactions

Nursing Considerations:

- Assess pain and inflammation levels.

- Monitor blood pressure and renal function.

- Caution in patients with cardiovascular disease.

Administration: Can be taken with or without food, but taking it with food may reduce gastrointestinal irritation.

Additional Information:

- Relatively lower risk of gastrointestinal bleeding compared to other NSAIDs.

CIPROFLOXACIN

Brand Names: Cipro

OTC Availability: No

Classification: Antibiotic (Fluoroquinolone Class)

Mechanism of Action: Inhibits bacterial DNA gyrase and topoisomerase IV, leading to bacterial cell death.

Indications:

- Urinary tract infections

- Respiratory infections

- Skin infections

Contraindications:

- Hypersensitivity to fluoroquinolones

- Concurrent use with tizanidine

- Pediatric patients (in some cases due to arthropathy)

Side Effects:
- Nausea

- Diarrhea

- Tendon rupture

- Photosensitivity

Nursing Considerations:
- Assess infection symptoms before and during treatment.

- Monitor for signs of tendonitis or tendon rupture.

- Instruct patients to avoid sun exposure and take with plenty of fluids.

- Be cautious in patients with renal impairment; dosage adjustment may be needed.

Additional Information:
- Risk of Clostridium difficile-associated diarrhea with broad-spectrum antibiotics like ciprofloxacin.

- May cause QT prolongation and should be used cautiously in patients with cardiac issues.

CITALOPRAM

Brand Names: Celexa

OTC Availability: No

Classification: Selective Serotonin Reuptake Inhibitor (SSRI)

Mechanism of Action: Inhibits the reuptake of serotonin, increasing its availability in the synaptic cleft.

Indications:

- Depression

- Anxiety disorders

Contraindications:

- Hypersensitivity to citalopram or related SSRIs

- Concurrent use of MAOIs

- QT prolongation

Side Effects:
- Nausea

- Insomnia

- Sexual dysfunction

- Increased suicidal thoughts

Nursing Considerations:
- Monitor mood and mental status.

- Assess for suicidal ideation.

Administration: Can be taken with or without food. Preferably, take it at the same time every day for best results.

Additional Information:
- Full therapeutic effects may take several weeks to manifest.

CLONAZEPAM

Brand Names: Klonopin

OTC Availability: No

Classification: Benzodiazepine

Mechanism of Action: Enhances the effect of GABA, a neurotransmitter, leading to sedation, muscle relaxation, and reduced anxiety.

Indications:
- Anxiety disorders
- Seizure disorders
- Panic disorders

Contraindications:

- Severe liver disorders

- Narrow-angle glaucoma

- Hypersensitivity to benzodiazepines

Side Effects:

- Drowsiness

- Impaired motor function

- Dependence

- Respiratory depression

Nursing Considerations:

- Assess anxiety and/or frequency of seizures.

- Monitor respiratory and central nervous system status.

Administration: Take it with or without food. If stomach upset occurs, take with food or milk.

Additional Information:

- Tapering off the medication is advised to avoid withdrawal symptoms.

CLOPIDOGREL

Brand Names: Plavix

OTC Availability: No

Classification: Antiplatelet

Mechanism of Action: Inhibits platelet aggregation by blocking the binding of ADP to its receptor on platelets.

Indications:

- Prevention of cardiovascular events

- After myocardial infarction

- Stroke

Contraindications:

- Active bleeding

- Hypersensitivity to clopidogrel

Side Effects:

- Bleeding

- Bruising

- Gastrointestinal upset

Nursing Considerations:

- Monitor for signs of bleeding.

- Check for history of bleeding disorders.

Administration: Can be taken with or without food.

Additional Information:

- May interact with other anticoagulants and certain other medications.

DIAZEPAM

Brand Names: Valium

OTC Availability: No

Classification: Benzodiazepine

Mechanism of Action: Enhances the effect of GABA, resulting in sedation, muscle relaxation, and anxiolytic effects.

Indications:

- Anxiety

- Muscle spasms

- Seizures

Contraindications:

- Severe respiratory depression

- Severe hepatic impairment

- Acute narrow-angle glaucoma

Side Effects:

- Drowsiness

- Respiratory depression

- Dependence

Nursing Considerations:

- Assess anxiety level and/or muscle spasm severity.

- Monitor respiratory status.

Administration: Can be taken with or without food. If stomach upset occurs, take with food.

Additional Information:

- Potential for abuse and dependence.

DICLOFENAC

Brand Names: Voltaren, Cataflam

OTC Availability: No

Classification: NSAID

Mechanism of Action: Inhibits COX enzymes, reducing inflammation and pain.

Indications:

- Acute and chronic pain

- Inflammation

Contraindications:

- Hypersensitivity to diclofenac or other NSAIDs

- History of gastrointestinal bleeding

Side Effects:

- Gastrointestinal bleeding

- Hepatic dysfunction

- Hypertension

Nursing Considerations:

- Assess pain and inflammation levels.

- Monitor liver function and blood pressure.

Administration: Should be taken with food to minimize gastrointestinal irritation.

Additional Information:

- Increased risk of cardiovascular events with prolonged use.

DONEPEZIL

Brand Names: Aricept

OTC Availability: No

Classification: Acetylcholinesterase Inhibitor

Mechanism of Action: Increases the concentration of acetylcholine in the brain by inhibiting its breakdown.

Indications:

- Alzheimer's Disease

- Dementia

Contraindications:

- Hypersensitivity to donepezil or piperidine derivatives

Side Effects:

- Nausea

- Diarrhea

- Insomnia

Nursing Considerations:

- Assess cognitive function regularly.

- Monitor for gastrointestinal side effects.

Administration: Take in the evening just before bed, with or without food.

Additional Information:

- Efficacy may be limited and is generally symptom-specific.

- Consult healthcare provider for regular follow-ups to assess efficacy and side effects.

DULOXETINE

Brand Names: Cymbalta, Drizalma Sprinkle

OTC Availability: No

Classification: SNRI (Serotonin-Norepinephrine Reuptake Inhibitor)

Mechanism of Action: Inhibits the reuptake of serotonin and norepinephrine.

Indications:

- Depression

- Generalized anxiety disorder

- Chronic pain conditions

Contraindications:

- Hypersensitivity to duloxetine

- Concurrent use with MAOIs

Side Effects:
- Nausea

- Dry mouth

- Sleep disturbances

Nursing Considerations:
- Monitor mood and mental status.

- Assess for suicidal ideation.

Administration: Should be taken with food to minimize nausea.

Additional Information:
- May increase blood pressure; monitor accordingly.

ENOXAPARIN

Brand Names: Lovenox

OTC Availability: No

Classification: Anticoagulant, Low-Molecular-Weight Heparin

Mechanism of Action: Inhibits clotting factors, preventing thrombus formation.

Indications:

- Deep vein thrombosis (DVT) prophylaxis

- Acute coronary syndrome

Contraindications:

- Active major bleeding

- Hypersensitivity to heparin or pork products

Side Effects:

- Bleeding

- Bruising

- Elevated liver enzymes

Nursing Considerations:

- Monitor for signs of bleeding.

- Periodically check coagulation levels.

Administration: Administered via subcutaneous injection. Do not mix with other injections.

Additional Information:

- Antidote is protamine sulfate.

ESCITALOPRAM

Brand Names: Lexapro

OTC Availability: No

Classification: SSRI (Selective Serotonin Reuptake Inhibitor)

Mechanism of Action: Increases the amount of serotonin available in the brain.

Indications:

- Depression

- Generalized anxiety disorder

Contraindications:

- Hypersensitivity to escitalopram or citalopram

- Concurrent use with MAOIs

Side Effects:

- Nausea

- Insomnia

- Sexual dysfunction

Nursing Considerations:

- Monitor mood and mental status.

- Assess for suicidal ideation.

Administration: Can be taken with or without food.

Additional Information:

- Tapering off is advised to avoid withdrawal symptoms.

FLUOXETINE

Brand Names: Prozac, Sarafem

OTC Availability: No

Classification: SSRI (Selective Serotonin Reuptake Inhibitor)

Mechanism of Action: Inhibits the reuptake of serotonin.

Indications:

- Depression

- Obsessive-compulsive disorder (OCD)

- Panic disorder

Contraindications:

- Hypersensitivity to fluoxetine

- Concurrent use with MAOIs

Side Effects:
- Nausea

- Sleep disturbances

- Sexual dysfunction

Nursing Considerations:
- Monitor mood and mental status.

- Assess for suicidal ideation.

Administration: Can be taken with or without food.

Additional Information:
- Long half-life; takes time to build up and taper off in the system.

FUROSEMIDE

Brand Names: Lasix

OTC Availability: No

Classification: Loop Diuretic

Mechanism of Action: Inhibits sodium and chloride reabsorption in the loop of Henle

Indications:

- Edema

- Hypertension

Contraindications:

- Anuria

- Hypersensitivity to sulfonamides

Side Effects:

- Dehydration

- Electrolyte imbalance

- Hypotension

Nursing Considerations:

- Monitor fluid and electrolyte status.

- Assess blood pressure and renal function.

Administration: Best taken in the morning to avoid nocturia.

Additional Information:

- Can increase risk of ototoxicity when taken with certain medications like aminoglycosides.

GABAPENTIN

Brand Names: Neurontin

OTC Availability: No

Classification: Anticonvulsant, Neuropathic Pain Agent

Mechanism of Action: Binds to calcium channels, reducing neuropathic pain and seizures.

Indications:

- Epilepsy

- Neuropathic pain

Contraindications:

- Hypersensitivity to gabapentin

Side Effects:

- Drowsiness

- Dizziness

- Peripheral edema

Nursing Considerations:

- Assess for pain level and/or seizure activity.

- Monitor for mood changes.

Administration: Can be taken with or without food, but consistency is advised for best absorption.

Additional Information:

- Tapering off is recommended to avoid withdrawal symptoms.

HALOPERIDOL

Brand Names: Haldol

OTC Availability: No

Classification: Typical Antipsychotic

Mechanism of Action: Blocks dopamine receptors in the brain.

Indications:

- Schizophrenia

- Acute agitation

- Tourette's syndrome

Contraindications:

- Severe CNS depression

- Parkinson's disease

Side Effects:

- Extrapyramidal symptoms

- Drowsiness

- Tardive dyskinesia

Nursing Considerations:

- Monitor for extrapyramidal symptoms.

- Assess mental status and agitation level.

Administration: Can be taken with or without food.

Additional Information:

- Antidote for severe extrapyramidal symptoms is diphenhy-
dramine or benztropine.

HYDROMORPHONE

Brand Names: Dilaudid, Exalgo

OTC Availability: No

Classification: Opioid Analgesic

Mechanism of Action: Binds to opioid receptors in the CNS, inhibiting pain pathways.

Indications:

- Moderate to severe pain

- Surgical analgesia

Contraindications:

- Hypersensitivity to hydromorphone

- Respiratory depression

Side Effects:

- Nausea

- Vomiting

- Respiratory depression

Nursing Considerations:

- Monitor respiratory rate and pain level.

- Assess for signs of opioid dependency.

Administration: Take with or without food; however, taking with food may minimize nausea.

Additional Information:

- High potential for abuse and dependency.

- Use caution with other CNS depressants.

HYDROCHLOROTHIAZIDE

Brand Names: Microzide, HydroDIURIL

OTC Availability: No

Classification: Thiazide Diuretic

Mechanism of Action: Inhibits sodium and chloride reabsorption in the distal convoluted tubule.

Indications:

- Hypertension

- Edema

Contraindications:

- Anuria

- Hypersensitivity to thiazides or sulfonamides

Side Effects:

- Electrolyte imbalance

- Dehydration

- Hypotension

Nursing Considerations:

- Monitor fluid and electrolyte status.

- Assess blood pressure.

Administration: Best taken in the morning to avoid nocturia.

Additional Information:

- May increase risk of gout.

Heparin

Brand Names: N/A

OTC Availability: No

Classification: Anticoagulant

Mechanism of Action: Inhibits clotting by enhancing antithrombin activity.

Indications:

- Prevention of thrombosis

- Treatment of existing clots

Contraindications:

- Active bleeding

- Hypersensitivity to heparin

Side Effects:

- Bleeding

- Thrombocytopenia

- Bruising

Nursing Considerations:

- Monitor for signs of bleeding.

- Regularly check coagulation levels (aPTT).

Administration: Intravenous or subcutaneous injection only.

Additional Information:

- Antidote is protamine sulfate.

IBUPROFEN

Brand Names: Advil, Motrin

OTC Availability: Yes (lower doses)

Classification: Nonsteroidal Anti-Inflammatory Drug (NSAID)

Mechanism of Action: Inhibits COX enzymes, leading to reduced production of prostaglandins, which in turn reduces inflammation, pain, and fever.

Indications:

- Mild to moderate pain

- Inflammation

- Fever

Contraindications:

- Hypersensitivity to ibuprofen or other NSAIDs

- History of gastrointestinal bleeding

- Severe renal impairment

Side Effects:
- Gastrointestinal bleeding

- Hypertension

- Kidney dysfunction

Nursing Considerations:
- Assess pain, inflammation, and/or fever levels.

- Monitor blood pressure and renal function.

- Caution in patients with cardiovascular disease.

Administration: Best taken with food or milk to minimize gastrointestinal irritation.

Additional Information:
- Increased risk of cardiovascular events with prolonged use.

- May interact with anticoagulants, certain antihypertensives, and other medications.

INSULIN

Brand Names: Varies by type (e.g., Humalog, NovoLog, Lantus)

OTC Availability: No

Classification: Hormone, Antidiabetic

Mechanism of Action: Lowers blood sugar by facilitating glucose uptake into cells.

Indications:

- Diabetes mellitus

Contraindications:

- Hypoglycemia

Side Effects:

- Hypoglycemia

- Weight gain

- Local injection site reactions

Nursing Considerations:
- Monitor blood glucose levels.

- Know onset, peak, and duration of the specific insulin type.

Administration: Subcutaneous injection or insulin pump; timing depends on the type of insulin.

Additional Information:
- Always double-check insulin type and dose.

LACTULOSE

Brand Names: Generlac, Enulose

OTC Availability: No

Classification: Osmotic Laxative

Mechanism of Action: Increases water content and softens the stool.

Indications:

- Constipation

- Hepatic encephalopathy

Contraindications:

- Bowel obstruction

Side Effects:

- Gas

- Cramping

- Diarrhea

Nursing Considerations:

- Monitor electrolyte levels for long-term use.

- Assess mental status when used for hepatic encephalopathy.

Administration: Oral; may be taken with or without food.

Levodopa/Carbidopa

Brand Names: Sinemet

OTC Availability: No

Classification: Dopamine Precursor / Decarboxylase Inhibitor

Mechanism of Action: Levodopa is converted to dopamine in the brain, while carbidopa prevents lev-

odopa from converting to dopamine outside of the brain.

Indications:

- Parkinson's disease

- Parkinson-like symptoms

Contraindications:

- Hypersensitivity to levodopa or carbidopa

- Narrow-angle glaucoma

Side Effects:

- Nausea

- Dizziness

- Dyskinesia

Nursing Considerations:

- Assess for 'on-off' phenomena.

- Monitor liver and kidney function.

Administration: Take on an empty stomach, at least 1 hour before or 2 hours after meals.

Additional Information:

- May cause drowsiness; caution when driving.

- May interact with MAO inhibitors.

LEVOTHYROXINE

Brand Names: Synthroid, Levoxyl

OTC Availability: No

Classification: Thyroid Hormone

Mechanism of Action: Synthetic form of thyroxine (T4), which increases metabolic rate.

Indications:

- Hypothyroidism

- Thyroid cancer

Contraindications:

- Untreated adrenal insufficiency

- Recent myocardial infarction

Side Effects:

- Tachycardia

- Insomnia

- Tremors

Nursing Considerations:

- Monitor thyroid function tests.

- Assess for signs of hyperthyroidism.

  Administration: Take on an empty stomach, 30-60 minutes before breakfast.

  Additional Information:

- Absorption is affected by food and certain medications like calcium and iron supplements.

LISINOPRIL

Brand Names: Prinivil, Zestril

OTC Availability: No

Classification: ACE Inhibitor

Mechanism of Action: Blocks the conversion of angiotensin I to angiotensin II, lowering blood pressure.

Indications:

- Hypertension

- Heart failure

Contraindications:

- Hypersensitivity to ACE inhibitors

- History of angioedema

Side Effects:

- Cough

- Elevated blood potassium levels

- Low blood pressure

Nursing Considerations:

- Monitor blood pressure and renal function.

- Assess for angioedema.

Administration: Best taken 1 hour before meals for better absorption.

Additional Information:

- May increase serum potassium levels; monitor accordingly.

LORAZEPAM

Brand Names: Ativan

OTC Availability: No

Classification: Benzodiazepine

Mechanism of Action: Enhances the effects of GABA, a neurotransmitter that inhibits brain activity.

Indications:

- Anxiety

- Insomnia

- Seizures

Contraindications:

- Hypersensitivity to benzodiazepines

- Acute narrow-angle glaucoma

Side Effects:

- Drowsiness

- Dizziness

- Respiratory depression

Nursing Considerations:

- Monitor mental status and respiratory function.

- Assess for signs of abuse.

Administration: With or without food; however, food may delay onset.

Additional Information:

- Risk of dependence; taper off gradually.

MEMANTINE

Brand Names: Namenda

OTC Availability: No

Classification: NMDA Receptor Antagonist

Mechanism of Action: Blocks the effects of excessive levels of glutamate, a neurotransmitter, that may lead to neuronal damage.

Indications:

- Moderate to severe Alzheimer's disease

Contraindications:

- Hypersensitivity to memantine

Side Effects:

- Dizziness

- Confusion

- Headache

Nursing Considerations:
- Assess cognitive function.

- Monitor for CNS changes, like hallucinations.

Administration: Take with or without food.

Additional Information:
- Not a cure for Alzheimer's; it may help with the symptoms.

- May interact with other NMDA antagonists or medications affecting renal function.

Menthol

Brand Names: Biofreeze, Bengay, Vicks VapoRub, among others

OTC or Prescription: Yes

Classification:

Topical analgesic, Decongestant

Mechanism of Action:

Menthol stimulates cold receptors in the skin, providing a cooling sensation. It also has mild local anesthetic properties.

Indications:

For temporary relief of minor aches and pains of muscles and joints, cough suppression, and nasal congestion.

Contraindications:

Hypersensitivity to menthol or any of the components in the product.

Side Effects:

Skin irritation, allergic reactions, eye irritation if contact occurs.

Nursing Considerations:

- Assess the affected area before application.

- Wash hands thoroughly before and after applying the topical menthol.

- Use only as directed and avoid application to broken or irritated skin.

- For external use only; avoid contact with eyes and mucous membranes.

Administration:

Generally, it can be applied up to 3-4 times daily. Apply a thin layer to the affected area and rub in gently until fully absorbed.

METOPROLOL

Brand Names: Lopressor, Toprol-XL

OTC Availability: No

Classification: Beta-Blocker

Mechanism of Action: Blocks β1-adrenergic receptors, lowering heart rate and blood pressure.

Indications:

- Hypertension

- Angina

- Heart failure

Contraindications:

- Severe bradycardia

- Heart block greater than first degree

Side Effects:

- Dizziness

- Bradycardia

- Fatigue

Nursing Considerations:

- Monitor heart rate and blood pressure.

- Assess for signs of heart failure.

Administration: Can be taken with or without food, but consistency is advised for best absorption.

Additional Information:

- Abrupt cessation may exacerbate angina or induce myocardial infarction.

METFORMIN

Brand Names: Glucophage

OTC Availability: No

Classification: Biguanide, Antidiabetic

Mechanism of Action: Decreases hepatic glucose production and improves insulin sensitivity.

Indications:

- Type 2 Diabetes

Contraindications:

- Renal impairment

- Severe infection

Side Effects:

- Nausea

- Diarrhea

- Lactic acidosis (rare)

Nursing Considerations:

- Monitor blood glucose and renal function.

- Assess for signs of lactic acidosis.

Administration: Take with meals to reduce gastrointestinal effects.

Additional Information:

- Alcohol increases the risk of lactic acidosis.

METHOTREXATE

Brand Names: Trexall, Rheumatrex

OTC Availability: No

Classification: Antimetabolite, Disease-Modifying Antirheumatic Drug (DMARD)

Mechanism of Action: Inhibits folic acid synthesis, reducing inflammation and slowing down the progression of arthritis.

Indications:

- Rheumatoid arthritis

- Psoriatic arthritis

Contraindications:

- Pregnancy

- Liver disease

- Immunodeficiency

Side Effects:
- Nausea

- Hair loss

- Liver toxicity

Nursing Considerations:
- Monitor liver and kidney function.

- Assess for signs of infection.

Administration: Take on an empty stomach, either 1 hour before or 2 hours after meals.

Additional Information:
- May require supplemental folic acid.

- Regular blood tests are essential for monitoring toxicity.

METRONIDAZOLE

Brand Names: Flagyl

OTC Availability: No

Classification: Antibiotic, Antiprotozoal

Mechanism of Action: Disrupts bacterial and protozoal DNA synthesis.

Indications:

- Bacterial vaginosis

- Trichomoniasis

- Anaerobic bacterial infections

Contraindications:

- Hypersensitivity to metronidazole

- First trimester of pregnancy

Side Effects:

- Nausea

- Metallic taste

- Peripheral neuropathy

Nursing Considerations:

- Monitor liver function tests.

- Assess for signs of superinfection.

Administration: Take with food to minimize gastrointestinal side effects.

Additional Information:

- Avoid alcohol during treatment and for at least 48 hours after completing the medication due to potential for a disulfiram-like reaction.

Mirtazapine

Brand Names: Remeron

OTC Availability: No

Classification: Antidepressant

Mechanism of Action: Increases the release of norepinephrine and serotonin.

Indications:

- Major depressive disorder

Contraindications:

- Hypersensitivity to mirtazapine

Side Effects:

- Drowsiness

- Weight gain

- Dry mouth

Nursing Considerations:

- Monitor mental status.

- Assess for signs of suicidal ideation.

Administration: Take with or without food; however, taking it with food may enhance absorption.

Additional Information:

- May cause serotonin syndrome when combined with other serotonergic agents.

Morphine

Brand Names: MS Contin, Kadian

OTC Availability: No

Classification: Opioid Analgesic

Mechanism of Action: Binds to opioid receptors, inhibiting the perception of pain.

Indications:

- Moderate to severe pain

Contraindications:

- Respiratory depression

- Hypersensitivity to opioids

Side Effects:

- Constipation

- Respiratory depression

- Drowsiness

Nursing Considerations:

- Monitor respiratory rate and signs of sedation.

- Assess pain level regularly.

Administration: With or without food, but if taken with food, maintain consistency.

Additional Information:

- Naloxone is the antidote for opioid overdose.

METHYL SALICYLATE

Brand Names: Bengay, Deep Heating

OTC Availability: Yes

Classification: Topical NSAID

Mechanism of Action: Produces heat to alleviate pain and has mild anti-inflammatory effects.

Indications:

- Muscle aches

- Joint pains

Contraindications:

- Hypersensitivity to salicylates or aspirin

Side Effects:

- Burning

- Irritation

Nursing Considerations:

- Apply to affected area as needed.

- Avoid broken skin.

Administration: Topical; apply to affected area no more than 3-4 times daily.

Naproxen

Brand Names: Aleve, Naprosyn

OTC Availability: Yes (lower strength)

Classification: Nonsteroidal Anti-Inflammatory Drug (NSAID)

Mechanism of Action: Inhibits COX enzymes, reducing inflammation.

Indications:

- Pain

- Inflammation

Contraindications:

- Peptic ulcer disease

- Hypersensitivity to NSAIDs

Side Effects:

- Gastrointestinal bleeding

- Headache

- Hypertension

Nursing Considerations:

- Monitor for signs of gastrointestinal bleeding.

- Assess pain and inflammation.

Administration: Take with food or milk to reduce gastrointestinal irritation.

Additional Information:

- Risk of cardiovascular events increases with prolonged use.

OMEPRAZOLE

Brand Names: Prilosec

OTC Availability: Yes

Classification: Proton Pump Inhibitor

Mechanism of Action: Inhibits gastric acid secretion.

Indications:

- Gastroesophageal reflux disease (GERD)

- Peptic ulcers

Contraindications:

- Hypersensitivity to omeprazole

Side Effects:

- Headache

- Nausea

- Diarrhea

Nursing Considerations:
- Monitor for signs of gastrointestinal bleeding.

- Assess for relief of symptoms.

Administration: Take 30 minutes before meals.

Additional Information:
- May interfere with absorption of certain medications requiring acidic environment.

Oxycodone

Brand Names: OxyContin, Percocet

OTC Availability: No

Classification: Opioid Analgesic

Mechanism of Action: Binds to opioid receptors to decrease perception of pain.

Indications:

- Moderate to severe pain

Contraindications:

- Respiratory depression

- Hypersensitivity to opioids

Side Effects:

- Constipation

- Respiratory depression

- Drowsiness

Nursing Considerations:
- Monitor respiratory rate and signs of sedation.

- Assess pain level regularly.

Administration: With or without food; if taken with food, maintain consistency.

Additional Information:
- Naloxone is the antidote for opioid overdose.

PANTOPRAZOLE

Brand Names: Protonix

OTC Availability: No

Classification: Proton Pump Inhibitor

Mechanism of Action: Inhibits gastric acid secretion.

Indications:

- Gastroesophageal reflux disease (GERD)

- Zollinger-Ellison syndrome

Contraindications:

- Hypersensitivity to pantoprazole

Side Effects:

- Diarrhea

- Headache

- Abdominal pain

Nursing Considerations:
- Monitor for signs of gastrointestinal bleeding.

- Assess for relief of symptoms.

Administration: Take 30 minutes before meals.

Additional Information:
- May interfere with the absorption of medications requiring an acidic environment.

POLYETHYLENE GLYCOL 3350

Brand Names: RestoraLAX, MiraLAX

OTC Availability: Yes

Classification: Osmotic Laxative

Mechanism of Action: Retains water in the stool, increasing stool volume which triggers bowel movement.

Indications:

- Constipation

Contraindications:

- Bowel obstruction

Side Effects:

- Bloating

- Cramping

- Gas

Nursing Considerations:

- Assess bowel function.

- Adequate hydration is important.

Administration: Oral; mix with a beverage and drink.

PROPRANOLOL

Brand Names: Inderal

OTC Availability: No

Classification: Beta-Blocker

Mechanism of Action: Blocks $\beta 1$ and $\beta 2$ adrenergic receptors, reducing heart rate and blood pressure.

Indications:

- Hypertension

- Angina

- Migraine prophylaxis

Contraindications:

- Severe bradycardia

- Heart block greater than first degree

Side Effects:

- Dizziness

- Bradycardia

- Fatigue

Nursing Considerations:

- Monitor heart rate and blood pressure.

- Assess for signs of heart failure.

Administration: Can be taken with or without food, but consistency is advised for best absorption.

Additional Information:

- Abrupt cessation may exacerbate angina or induce myocardial infarction.

PREDNISONE

Brand Names: Deltasone

OTC Availability: No

Classification: Corticosteroid

Mechanism of Action: Anti-inflammatory and immunosuppressive effects.

Indications:

- Asthma

- Autoimmune diseases

- Allergic reactions

Contraindications:

- Fungal infections

- Hypersensitivity to prednisone

Side Effects:
- Weight gain

- Osteoporosis

- Hyperglycemia

Nursing Considerations:
- Monitor blood glucose levels.

- Assess for signs of infection.

Administration: Take with food or milk to reduce gastrointestinal irritation.

Additional Information:
- Abrupt cessation can lead to adrenal insufficiency.

QUETIAPINE

Brand Names: Seroquel

OTC Availability: No

Classification: Atypical Antipsychotic

Mechanism of Action: Blocks dopamine and serotonin receptors in the brain.

Indications:

- Schizophrenia

- Bipolar disorder

- Depression

Contraindications:

- Hypersensitivity to quetiapine

Side Effects:

- Drowsiness

- Weight gain

- Dry mouth

Nursing Considerations:

- Monitor for extrapyramidal symptoms.

- Assess mental status.
  Administration: Take with or without food; if taken with food, maintain consistency.
  Additional Information:

- Increased risk of death in elderly patients with dementia-related psychosis.

RISPERIDONE

Brand Names: Risperdal

OTC Availability: No

Classification: Atypical Antipsychotic

Mechanism of Action: Blocks dopamine and serotonin receptors in the brain.

Indications:

- Schizophrenia

- Bipolar disorder

Contraindications:

- Hypersensitivity to risperidone

Side Effects:

- Drowsiness

- Weight gain

- Extrapyramidal symptoms

Nursing Considerations:

- Monitor for extrapyramidal symptoms.

- Assess mental status.

Administration: Take with or without food; if taken with food, maintain consistency.

Additional Information:

- Increased risk of death in elderly patients with dementia-related psychosis.

RIVASTIGMINE

Brand Names: Exelon

OTC or Prescription: Yes

Classification:

Cholinesterase inhibitor

Mechanism of Action:

Inhibits acetylcholinesterase, an enzyme that breaks down acetylcholine, thus increasing the levels of acetylcholine in the brain. This is thought to improve the symptoms of dementia.

Indications:

Used primarily for the treatment of mild to moderate Alzheimer's disease and Parkinson's disease dementia.

Contraindications:

- Known hypersensitivity to rivastigmine or similar medications.

- Severe liver impairment.

Side Effects:

- Nausea

- Vomiting

- Loss of appetite

- Dizziness

- Weakness

Nursing Considerations:

- Monitor for adverse gastrointestinal effects, especially during initial therapy.

- Assess cognitive function routinely to determine medication efficacy.

- Be cautious with patients having a history of asthma or obstructive pulmonary diseases.

Administration:

Rivastigmine is available in both oral forms and a transdermal patch. For the oral route, it is usually advised to take it with meals. The patch is generally applied once a day; follow specific guidelines for application.

RANITIDINE

Brand Names: Zantac

OTC Availability: Previously available, but withdrawn from market due to safety concerns

Classification: H2 Receptor Antagonist

Mechanism of Action: Blocks histamine at H2 receptors in stomach, reducing acid production.

Indications:

- Peptic ulcer

- GERD

Contraindications:

- Hypersensitivity to ranitidine

Side Effects:

- Headache

- Diarrhea

- Fatigue

Nursing Considerations:

- Monitor for signs of gastrointestinal bleeding.

- Assess for relief of symptoms.

Administration: Take 30 minutes before meals.

Additional Information:

- Has been withdrawn in many regions due to concerns over potential carcinogenic impurities.

SIMVASTATIN

Brand Names: Zocor

OTC Availability: No

Classification: HMG-CoA Reductase Inhibitor (Statin)

Mechanism of Action: Inhibits cholesterol synthesis in liver.

Indications:

- Hypercholesterolemia

- Cardiovascular risk reduction

Contraindications:

- Liver disease

- Hypersensitivity to simvastatin

Side Effects:

- Myalgia

- Elevated liver enzymes

- Headache

Nursing Considerations:

- Monitor liver function tests.

- Assess lipid levels.

Administration: Take in the evening, either with or without food.

Additional Information:

- Risk of myopathy increases with higher doses or concurrent use of certain medications.

SENNOSIDES

Brand Names: Senokot, Ex-Lax

OTC Availability: Yes

Classification: Stimulant Laxative

Mechanism of Action: Stimulates the lining of the bowel to promote peristalsis, facilitating bowel movements.

Indications:

- Constipation

Contraindications:

- Bowel obstruction

- Hypersensitivity to senna or any component

Side Effects:

- Abdominal cramps

- Diarrhea

- Nausea

Nursing Considerations:

- Assess bowel function.

- Use should be short-term unless directed by a healthcare provider.

Administration: Oral, usually before bed; can be taken with or without food.

Additional Information:

- Onset of action is usually 6 to 12 hours after administration.

- Not recommended for prolonged use without medical supervision.

SERTRALINE

Brand Names: Zoloft

OTC Availability: No

Classification: Selective Serotonin Reuptake Inhibitor (SSRI)

Mechanism of Action: Increases serotonin levels in the brain.

Indications:

- Depression

- Generalized Anxiety Disorder

- Obsessive-Compulsive Disorder

Contraindications:

- Concurrent use with MAOIs

- Hypersensitivity to sertraline

Side Effects:

- Nausea

- Insomnia

- Sexual dysfunction

Nursing Considerations:

- Monitor for worsening depression or suicidality.

- Assess mental status.
  Administration: Take with food to minimize gastrointestinal side effects.

Additional Information:

- Gradual dose tapering is recommended upon discontinuation.

SULFAMETHOXAZOLE/TRIME

Brand Names: Bactrim, Septra

OTC Availability: No

Classification: Antibiotic (Sulfonamide)

Mechanism of Action: Inhibits bacterial folic acid synthesis.

Indications:

- Urinary Tract Infections

- Respiratory Infections

- Skin Infections

Contraindications:

- Severe renal or hepatic dysfunction

- Hypersensitivity to sulfonamides

Side Effects:

- Rash

- Nausea

- Hyperkalemia

Nursing Considerations:

- Monitor renal function.

- Encourage fluid intake to prevent crystal formation.

Administration: Take with or without food, but with a full glass of water.

Additional Information:

- Avoid in late pregnancy and breastfeeding.

Tamsulosin

Brand Names: Flomax

OTC Availability: No

Classification: Alpha-1 Adrenergic Blocker

Mechanism of Action: Relaxes smooth muscle in the prostate and bladder neck.

Indications:

- Benign Prostatic Hyperplasia (BPH)

Contraindications:

- Hypersensitivity to tamsulosin

Side Effects:

- Dizziness

- Orthostatic hypotension

- Nasal congestion

Nursing Considerations:
- Monitor for signs of hypotension.

- Assess urinary symptoms.

Administration: Take 30 minutes after the same meal each day.

Additional Information:
- Risk of floppy iris syndrome in cataract surgery.

Venlafaxine

Brand Names: Effexor

OTC Availability: No

Classification: Serotonin-Norepinephrine Reuptake Inhibitor (SNRI)

Mechanism of Action: Increases levels of serotonin and norepinephrine in the brain.

Indications:

- Depression

- Generalized Anxiety Disorder

- Panic Disorder

Contraindications:

- Concurrent use with MAOIs

- Hypersensitivity to venlafaxine

Side Effects:
- Nausea

- Insomnia

- Hypertension

Nursing Considerations:
- Monitor blood pressure.

- Assess for worsening depression or suicidality.

Administration: Take with food to reduce gastrointestinal side effects.

Additional Information:
- Gradual dose tapering is recommended upon discontinuation.

PROPER ADMINISTRATION OF INHALERS

Twelve Rights of Medication Administration

1. **Right Patient**: Confirm the patient's identity using at least two identifiers, like name and date of birth.

2. **Right Medication and Expiration**: Double-check the medication against the prescription. Make sure it has not expired.

3. **Right Dose**: Measure the prescribed dose carefully, using the appropriate instrument.

4. **Right Route**: Confirm that the medication should be given via the intended route (oral, IV, etc.).

5. **Right Time**: Administer the medication at the time prescribed.

6. **Right Documentation**: Record all pertinent information, including medication, dose, time, and any patient reactions.

7. **Right Reason**: Understand the reason for the medication and educate the patient as necessary.

8. **Right to Refuse**: Acknowledge that the patient has the right to refuse medication; their decision should be respected and documented.

9. **Right Response**: Monitor the patient for the expected effects and any possible side effects.

10. **Right Education**: Provide necessary education to the patient or caregiver about the medication.

11. **Right Evaluation**: After administration, evaluate the patient's response to the medication, both therapeutically and for any adverse reactions.

12. **Right to Know**: Ensure the patient and their caregivers understand what medication is being administered, why it is being administered, and what the potential side effects may be.

Step-by-Step Guide to Administering an Inhaler

1. **Hand Hygiene**: First, wash your hands thoroughly with soap and water or use hand sanitizer.

2. **Check Inhaler**: Examine the inhaler for any visible damage. Make sure it contains sufficient medication and check the

expiration date.

3. **Prepare the Inhaler**: Remove the cap from the inhaler mouthpiece and shake the inhaler well.

4. **Position**: Stand or sit up straight to allow for full lung expansion.

5. **Breath Control**: Instruct the patient to exhale fully to empty the lungs of air.

6. **Mouthpiece Placement**: Place the mouthpiece between your lips and close your lips around it to form a seal. Alternatively, use a spacer if available and recommended.

7. **Inhalation**: Instruct the patient to start inhaling slowly through their mouth. As they do, press down on the inhaler to release one puff of medication. Continue to inhale deeply and slowly.

8. **Breath Hold**: After inhalation, hold the breath for about 10 seconds or as long as comfortably possible to allow the medication to settle in the lungs.

9. **Exhale**: Exhale slowly through the nose or mouth.

10. **Repeat**: If more than one puff is prescribed, wait about 1 minute between puffs and repeat steps 3 to 9.

11. **Cap and Store**: Replace the cap on the inhaler and store it in a cool, dry place.

Instructions for the Patient

- Make sure you know how many doses are remaining in your inhaler and replace it as needed.

- Rinse your mouth with water after using certain types of inhalers, as advised by your healthcare provider, to reduce the risk of oral infections.

- Consistently use your inhaler as prescribed, and do not skip doses.

- Always bring your inhaler with you in case of emergencies.

- If you experience any side effects or have difficulty using the inhaler, consult your healthcare provider.

FLUTICASONE

Brand Names: Flovent

OTC Availability: No

Classification: Corticosteroid

Mechanism of Action: Reduces inflammation in the airways.

Indications:

- Asthma

- Chronic obstructive pulmonary disease (COPD)

Contraindications:

- Hypersensitivity to fluticasone

Side Effects:

- Throat irritation

- Hoarseness

- Oral candidiasis (thrush)

Nursing Considerations:
- Assess lung function.

- Instruct on proper inhaler technique.

Administration: Inhale through the mouth; rinse mouth after use to prevent oral thrush.

Additional Information:
- Not for relief of acute bronchospasm.

- Requires regular use for maximum benefit.

SALMETEROL

Brand Names: Serevent

OTC Availability: No

Classification: Long-Acting Beta2-Agonist (LABA)

Mechanism of Action: Dilates the bronchial airways by acting on beta2 receptors.

Indications:

- Asthma

- COPD

Contraindications:

- Hypersensitivity to salmeterol

Side Effects:

- Headache

- Tremor

- Palpitations

Nursing Considerations:

- Monitor for increased use of short-acting beta2-agonists.

- Assess for paradoxical bronchospasm.

Administration: Inhale through the mouth.

Additional Information:

- Not for relief of acute symptoms.

- Generally used with an inhaled corticosteroid.

BUDESONIDE

Brand Names: Pulmicort

OTC Availability: No

Classification: Corticosteroid

Mechanism of Action: Reduces airway inflammation.

Indications:

- Asthma

  Contraindications:

- Hypersensitivity to budesonide

Side Effects:

- Oral candidiasis (thrush)

- Throat irritation

- Hoarseness

Nursing Considerations:

- Assess lung function.

- Instruct on proper inhaler technique.

Administration: Inhale through the mouth; rinse mouth after use to prevent oral thrush.

Additional Information:

- Requires regular use for full benefit.

- Not for relief of acute bronchospasm.

Ipratropium Bromide

Brand Names: Atrovent

OTC Availability: No

Classification: Anticholinergic Bronchodilator

Mechanism of Action: Blocks acetylcholine in the airways, leading to bronchodilation.

Indications:

- COPD

- Asthma

Contraindications:

- Hypersensitivity to ipratropium or atropine derivatives

Side Effects:

- Dry mouth

- Cough

- Headache

Nursing Considerations:

- Assess lung function.

- Monitor for anticholinergic side effects.

Administration: Inhale through the mouth.

Additional Information:

- Not for the treatment of acute bronchospasm.

- Can be used in combination with other bronchodilators for added effect.

Beclomethasone

Brand Names: Qvar

OTC Availability: No

Classification: Corticosteroid

Mechanism of Action: Reduces airway inflammation.

Indications:

- Asthma

Contraindications:

- Hypersensitivity to beclomethasone

Side Effects:

- Oral candidiasis (thrush)

- Hoarseness

- Throat irritation

Nursing Considerations:

- Assess lung function.

- Instruct on proper inhaler technique.

Administration: Inhale through the mouth; rinse mouth after use to prevent oral thrush.

Additional Information:

- Requires regular use for full benefit.

- Not for relief of acute bronchospasm.

MOMETASONE

Brand Names: Asmanex

OTC Availability: No

Classification: Corticosteroid

Mechanism of Action: Reduces airway inflammation.

Indications:

- Asthma

Contraindications:

- Hypersensitivity to mometasone

Side Effects:

- Oral candidiasis (thrush)

- Headache

- Sore throat

Nursing Considerations:
- Assess lung function.

- Instruct on proper inhaler technique.

Administration: Inhale through the mouth; rinse mouth after use to prevent oral thrush.

Additional Information:
- Not for relief of acute bronchospasm.

- Requires regular use for full benefit.

FORMOTEROL

Brand Names: Foradil, Oxeze

OTC Availability: No

Classification: Long-Acting Beta2-Agonist (LABA)

Mechanism of Action: Dilates the bronchial airways by acting on beta2 receptors.

Indications:

- Asthma

- COPD

Contraindications:

- Hypersensitivity to formoterol

Side Effects:

- Palpitations

- Tremor

- Insomnia

Nursing Considerations:

- Monitor for increased use of short-acting beta2-agonists.

- Assess for paradoxical bronchospasm.

Administration: Inhale through the mouth.

Additional Information:

- Not for relief of acute symptoms.

- Generally used with an inhaled corticosteroid.

CICLESONIDE

Brand Names: Alvesco

OTC Availability: No

Classification: Corticosteroid

Mechanism of Action: Reduces inflammation in the airways.

Indications:

- Asthma

Contraindications:

- Hypersensitivity to ciclesonide

Side Effects:

- Oral candidiasis (thrush)

- Throat irritation

- Hoarseness

Nursing Considerations:
- Assess lung function.

- Instruct on proper inhaler technique.

Administration: Inhale through the mouth; rinse mouth after use to prevent oral thrush.

Additional Information:
- Not for relief of acute bronchospasm.

- Requires regular use for full benefit.

TIOTROPIUM

Brand Names: Spiriva

OTC Availability: No

Classification: Anticholinergic Bronchodilator

Mechanism of Action: Blocks acetylcholine in the airways, leading to bronchodilation.

Indications:

- COPD

- Asthma

Contraindications:

- Hypersensitivity to tiotropium or atropine derivatives

Side Effects:

- Dry mouth

- Constipation

- Urinary retention

Nursing Considerations:

- Assess lung function.

- Monitor for anticholinergic side effects.

Administration: Inhale through the mouth.

Additional Information:

- Not for relief of acute bronchospasm.

- Long-term maintenance medication.

SALBUTAMOL

Brand Names:

Ventolin, ProAir, Albuterol (in the United States)

OTC or Prescription:

Prescription Only

Classification: Bronchodilator, Beta-2 Agonist

Mechanism of Action:

Activates beta-2 adrenergic receptors in the lungs, leading to relaxation of bronchial smooth muscles. This widens the airways, making breathing easier.

Indications:

- Asthma

- Chronic obstructive pulmonary disease (COPD)

- Exercise-induced bronchoconstriction

Contraindications:

- Hypersensitivity to Salbutamol or other beta-2 agonists

- Certain heart conditions without physician approval

Side Effects:

- Tremors

- Nervousness

- Rapid heart rate

- Palpitations

Nursing Considerations:

- Monitor lung function (e.g., peak flow).

- Assess for signs of paradoxical bronchospasm (worsening breathing).

- Educate the patient on proper inhaler technique.

Administration:

- **Inhaler:**

  - Shake well before use.

- Exhale fully and place mouthpiece in mouth.

- As you start to inhale, press down on the inhaler.

- Hold breath for about 10 seconds, then exhale.

- Wait at least 1 minute between puffs.

- Rinse mouth after use to prevent oral thrush.

Indacaterol

Brand Names: Onbrez

OTC Availability: No

Classification: Long-Acting Beta2-Agonist (LABA)

Mechanism of Action: Dilates the bronchial airways by acting on beta2 receptors.

Indications:

- COPD

Contraindications:

- Hypersensitivity to indacaterol

Side Effects:

- Palpitations

- Tremor

- Insomnia

Nursing Considerations:

- Monitor for increased use of short-acting beta2-agonists.

- Assess for paradoxical bronchospasm.

Administration: Inhale through the mouth.

Additional Information:

- Not for relief of acute symptoms.

- Generally not recommended for asthma.

VILANTEROL

Brand Names: Anoro, Breo

OTC Availability: No

Classification: Long-Acting Beta2-Agonist (LABA)

Mechanism of Action: Dilates the bronchial airways by acting on beta2 receptors.

Indications:

- COPD

Contraindications:

- Hypersensitivity to vilanterol

Side Effects:

- Palpitations

- Tremor

- Insomnia

Nursing Considerations:
- Monitor for increased use of short-acting beta2-agonists.

- Assess for paradoxical bronchospasm.

Administration: Inhale through the mouth.

Additional Information:
- Not for relief of acute symptoms.

- Often combined with other medications like fluticasone.

Olodaterol

Brand Names: Striverdi Respimat

OTC Availability: No

Classification: Long-Acting Beta-Agonist (LABA)

Mechanism of Action: Acts on beta-2 receptors in the bronchial smooth muscle, causing bronchodilation.

Indications:

- Maintenance treatment of airflow obstruction in patients with chronic obstructive pulmonary disease (COPD)

Contraindications:

- Not for treatment of asthma without the use of a long-term asthma control medication

- Acute bronchospasm

Side Effects:
- Dry mouth

- Upper respiratory tract infection

- Cough

Nursing Considerations:
- Assess respiratory function regularly.

- Not to be used as a rescue inhaler.

- Monitor for signs of paradoxical bronchospasm.

Administration: Inhalation; usually one inhalation (2.5 mcg) once daily.

Additional Information:
- Inhaler contains 60 doses, enough for one month of medication.

- Should not be used more than once in 24 hours.

PROPER APPLICATION OF HEMORRHOID CREAM

Twelve Rights of Medication Administration

1. **Right Patient**: Confirm the patient's identity using at least two identifiers, like name and date of birth.

2. **Right Medication and Expiration**: Double-check the medication against the prescription. Make sure it has not expired.

3. **Right Dose**: Measure the prescribed dose carefully, using the appropriate instrument.

4. **Right Route**: Confirm that the medication should be given via the intended route (oral, IV, etc.).

5. **Right Time**: Administer the medication at the time prescribed.

6. **Right Documentation**: Record all pertinent information, including medication, dose, time, and any patient reactions.

7. **Right Reason**: Understand the reason for the medication and educate the patient as necessary.

8. **Right to Refuse**: Acknowledge that the patient has the right to refuse medication; their decision should be respected and documented.

9. **Right Response**: Monitor the patient for the expected effects and any possible side effects.

10. **Right Education**: Provide necessary education to the patient or caregiver about the medication.

11. **Right Evaluation**: After administration, evaluate the patient's response to the medication, both therapeutically and for any adverse reactions.

12. **Right to Know**: Ensure the patient and their caregivers understand what medication is being administered, why it is being administered, and what the potential side effects may be.

1. **Preparation:**

   - Verify the prescription, confirming the drug, dose, and frequency according to the "12 Rights of Medication Administration."

   - Wash your hands thoroughly.

- If the patient is not yourself, explain the process to the patient and ensure they are in a comfortable position.

2. Site Cleansing:

- Gently clean the anal area with mild soap and water or use a moistened wipe.

- Pat the area dry with a soft towel; do not rub or use tissue paper that might worsen irritation.

3. Cream Preparation:

- Remove the cap of the cream tube.

- If the cream comes with an applicator, attach it to the tube as per the manufacturer's instructions.

4. Application:

- Apply a small amount of the cream to your finger or the applicator, depending on how the medication is meant to be applied.

- Gently apply the cream to the affected area around the outside of the anus or insert into the rectum as per instructions.

- If an applicator is used, clean it thoroughly after each application.

5. Hand Washing:

- Wash your hands thoroughly after application.

6. **Documentation:**

- Record the application in the medical record, noting the time and any patient comments if you are a healthcare provider.

7. **Monitoring:**

- Monitor for therapeutic effects and potential side effects.

- Instruct the patient to report any continued irritation, bleeding, or lack of symptom improvement.

Hydrocortisone

Brand Names: Anusol-HC, Proctozone

OTC Availability: Yes (Lower strength)

Classification: Topical Corticosteroid

Mechanism of Action: Reduces inflammation, itching, and swelling.

Indications:
- Hemorrhoids

Contraindications:
- Fungal, viral, or bacterial infections of the anal area

Side Effects:

- Burning

- Itching

- Dry skin

Nursing Considerations:
- Assess severity and extent of hemorrhoids.

- Do not use for prolonged periods without medical advice.

Administration: Topical; apply to affected area as directed, usually 2-4 times daily.

Additional Information:
- Wash hands before and after application.

- Avoid excessive use as it may lead to skin thinning.

PHENYLEPHRINE TOPICAL

Brand Names: Preparation H

OTC Availability: Yes

Classification: Vasoconstrictor

Mechanism of Action: Constricts blood vessels in the affected area to reduce swelling.

Indications:

- Hemorrhoids

Contraindications:

- Hypersensitivity to phenylephrine

Side Effects:

- Mild burning or itching

- Dry skin

Nursing Considerations:
- Assess the affected area before and during treatment.

- Use should be short-term unless directed by healthcare provider.

Administration: Topical; apply to the affected area as directed, usually up to 4 times daily.

Additional Information:
- Not to be ingested; for external use only.

- Wash hands before and after application.

ZINC OXIDE

Brand Names:

Desitin, Balmex, Calmoseptine (among others)

OTC or Prescription:

Over-The-Counter (OTC)

Classification:

Skin Protectant, Astringent

Mechanism of Action:

Forms a physical barrier on the skin to protect against moisture and irritants. It also has mild astringent and antiseptic properties.

Indications:

- Diaper rash

- Minor burns or skin irritation

- Sunscreen (in specific formulations)

Contraindications:

- Hypersensitivity to Zinc Oxide or other components

- Infected or deeply punctured skin (unless advised by a healthcare provider)

Side Effects:
- Rare, but may include local skin irritation

Nursing Considerations:
- Assess the skin area for signs of infection or irritation.

- Consult healthcare provider for deep or puncture wounds or serious burns.

Administration:
- **Topical Cream/Ointment:**

    ○ Clean the affected area gently.

    ○ Pat dry or allow to air dry.

    ○ Apply a thin layer of Zinc Oxide cream or ointment to the affected area as needed.

    ○ For diaper rash, apply during each diaper change, especially at bedtime or when exposure to wet diapers may be prolonged.

Proper Administration of Eye Drops

Twelve Rights of Medication Administration

1. **Right Patient**: Confirm the patient's identity using at least two identifiers, like name and date of birth.

2. **Right Medication and Expiration**: Double-check the medication against the prescription. Make sure it has not expired.

3. **Right Dose**: Measure the prescribed dose carefully, using the appropriate instrument.

4. **Right Route**: Confirm that the medication should be given via the intended route (oral, IV, etc.).

5. **Right Time**: Administer the medication at the time prescribed.

6. **Right Documentation**: Record all pertinent information, including medication, dose, time, and any patient reactions.

7. **Right Reason**: Understand the reason for the medication and educate the patient as necessary.

8. **Right to Refuse**: Acknowledge that the patient has the right to refuse medication; their decision should be respected and documented.

9. **Right Response**: Monitor the patient for the expected effects and any possible side effects.

10. **Right Education**: Provide necessary education to the patient or caregiver about the medication.

11. **Right Evaluation**: After administration, evaluate the patient's response to the medication, both therapeutically and for any adverse reactions.

12. **Right to Know**: Ensure the patient and their caregivers understand what medication is being administered, why it is being administered, and what the potential side effects may be.

Step-by-Step Guide to Administering Eye Drops

1. **Hand Hygiene**: Wash your hands thoroughly with soap and water or use hand sanitizer before touching the eye drop bottle or your eyes.

2. **Check Expiration and Contents**: Make sure the eye drop bottle is not expired and that it contains enough medication for the application.

3. **Prepare**: Shake the bottle if required by the instructions, and remove the bottle cap carefully.

4. **Position**: Tilt the head backward or lie down, looking up at the ceiling.

5. **Eyelid Manipulation**: Use one hand to gently pull down the lower eyelid to create a "pocket" for the drop.

6. **Hold Bottle Correctly**: Hold the bottle with the other hand, about an inch above the eye, taking care not to touch the eye or eyelashes.

7. **Squeeze**: Gently squeeze the bottle to let one drop fall into the eye pocket made by the lower eyelid. Do not blink immediately.

8. **Close Eye**: Close the eye for a few seconds (or minutes if instructed) without blinking, and gently press the inner corner of the eye with a finger to minimize systemic absorption of the medication.

9. **Wipe Excess**: Use a tissue to wipe away any excess medication on the eyelid or cheeks.

10. **Recap**: Immediately replace the bottle cap.

11. **Document**: If you are a healthcare provider, remember to document the medication administration.

Instructions for the Patient

- Store the eye drop bottle as instructed, usually in a cool, dry place.

- Follow the prescribed frequency and duration for using the eye drops.

- Never share eye drops with others.

- If you experience any side effects or discomfort, consult your healthcare provider immediately.

Artificial Tears (Lubricant Eye Drops)

Brand Names: Refresh, Systane, Blink, Optive

OTC Availability: Yes

Classification: Eye Lubricant

Mechanism of Action: Moisturizes and lubricates the eye surface.

Indications:

- Dry eyes

- Eye irritation

Contraindications:

- Eye infection

Side Effects:

- Mild burning or stinging

Nursing Considerations:

- Assess eye dryness and irritation.

- Ensure proper administration technique to avoid contamination.

Administration: Ophthalmic; as needed.

Additional Information:

- Use as directed or as often as needed.

- Discard single-use vials after use.

AZELASTINE

Brand Names: Optivar

OTC Availability: No

Classification: Antihistamine

Mechanism of Action: Blocks histamine receptors, reducing allergic reactions.

Indications:

- Allergic conjunctivitis

Contraindications:

- Hypersensitivity

Side Effects:

- Eye irritation

- Burning or stinging

Nursing Considerations:
- Monitor for worsening signs of allergy.

- Counsel on proper administration technique.

Administration: Ophthalmic; as prescribed, usually twice daily.

BRIMONIDINE

Brand Names: Alphagan P

OTC Availability: No

Classification: Alpha-2 Adrenergic Agonist

Mechanism of Action: Reduces intraocular pressure by decreasing aqueous humor production and increasing uveoscleral outflow.

Indications:

- Open-angle glaucoma

- Ocular hypertension

Contraindications:

- Hypersensitivity

Side Effects:

- Dry mouth

- Burning

- Stinging

Nursing Considerations:

- Assess intraocular pressure regularly.

- Monitor for signs of allergic reaction.

Administration: Ophthalmic; as prescribed, usually twice or thrice daily.

CIPROFLOXACIN

Brand Names: Ciloxan

OTC Availability: No

Classification: Fluoroquinolone Antibiotic

Mechanism of Action: Inhibits bacterial DNA gyrase, preventing bacterial DNA replication.

Indications:

- Bacterial conjunctivitis

- Corneal ulcers

Contraindications:

- Hypersensitivity

Side Effects:

- Eye irritation

- Blurred vision

Nursing Considerations:

- Monitor for signs of allergic reaction.

- Ensure proper hygiene to avoid cross-contamination.

Administration: Ophthalmic; as prescribed, often 4-6 times daily.

CYCLOPENTOLATE

Brand Names: Cyclogyl

OTC Availability: No

Classification: Mydriatic Agent

Mechanism of Action: Blocks the action of acetylcholine, causing dilation of the pupil.

Indications:

- Pupil dilation for diagnostic procedures

Contraindications:

- Glaucoma

- Hypersensitivity

Side Effects:

- Temporary blurred vision

- Eye irritation

Nursing Considerations:

- Monitor for signs of glaucoma.

- Warn patient about temporary vision changes.

Administration: Ophthalmic; as prescribed, usually 1-2 drops before exam.

DEXAMETHASONE

Brand Names: Maxidex

OTC Availability: No

Classification: Corticosteroid

Mechanism of Action: Reduces inflammation by inhibiting multiple inflammatory substances.

Indications:

- Eye inflammation

- Post-operative care

Contraindications:

- Viral eye infections

- Fungal eye infections

Side Effects:

- Eye discomfort

- Blurred vision

Nursing Considerations:

- Monitor for worsening signs of infection.

- Counsel on proper administration technique.

Administration: Ophthalmic; as prescribed, usually 4-6 times daily initially.

DORZOLAMIDE

Brand Names: Trusopt

OTC Availability: No

Classification: Carbonic Anhydrase Inhibitor

Mechanism of Action: Reduces intraocular pressure by inhibiting aqueous humor production.

Indications:

- Open-angle glaucoma

- Ocular hypertension

Contraindications:

- Hypersensitivity

Side Effects:

- Eye burning

- Stinging

Nursing Considerations:

- Monitor intraocular pressure.

- Avoid use with sulfonamide allergy

Administration: Ophthalmic; as prescribed, usually three times daily.

ERYTHROMYCIN

Brand Names: Ilotycin

OTC Availability: No

Classification: Macrolide Antibiotic

Mechanism of Action: Inhibits bacterial protein synthesis by binding to the 50S ribosomal subunit.

Indications:

- Bacterial conjunctivitis

- Prophylaxis for neonatal conjunctivitis

Contraindications:

- Hypersensitivity

Side Effects:

- Eye irritation

- Burning sensation

Nursing Considerations:

- Monitor for signs of worsening infection.

- Educate on proper hygiene to avoid cross-contamination.

Administration: Ophthalmic; as prescribed, usually 3-4 times daily.

Gentamicin

Brand Names: Garamycin, Genoptic

OTC Availability: No

Classification: Aminoglycoside Antibiotic

Mechanism of Action: Inhibits bacterial protein synthesis, leading to bacterial cell death.

Indications:

- Bacterial conjunctivitis

- Keratitis

Contraindications:

- Hypersensitivity

Side Effects:

- Eye irritation

- Stinging

Nursing Considerations:

- Monitor for signs of worsening infection.

- Educate on proper hygiene to avoid cross-contamination.

Administration: Ophthalmic; as prescribed, usually every 4 hours.

KETOROLAC

Brand Names: Acular, Toradol

OTC Availability: No

Classification: NSAID

Mechanism of Action: Inhibits prostaglandin synthesis, providing analgesic and anti-inflammatory effects.

Indications:

- Postoperative inflammation

Contraindications:

- Active bleeding

Side Effects:

- Stinging

- Burning

Nursing Considerations:

- Assess for signs of eye infection or damage.

- Do not use for prolonged periods.

Administration: Ophthalmic; as prescribed, usually 4 times daily.

Latanoprost

Brand Names: Xalatan

OTC Availability: No

Classification: Prostaglandin Analogue

Mechanism of Action: Increases the outflow of aqueous humor, reducing intraocular pressure.

Indications:

- Open-angle glaucoma

- Ocular hypertension

Contraindications:

- Hypersensitivity

Side Effects:
- Darkening of the iris

- Eye irritation

Nursing Considerations:
- Monitor intraocular pressure.

- Counsel patients on potential eye color change.

Administration: Ophthalmic; once daily in the evening.

Naphazoline

Brand Names: Clear Eyes, Naphcon

OTC Availability: Yes

Classification: Decongestant

Mechanism of Action: Constricts blood vessels in the eyes, reducing redness.

Indications:

- Eye redness

Contraindications:

- Narrow-angle glaucoma

- Hypersensitivity

Side Effects:

- Eye irritation

- Increased intraocular pressure

Nursing Considerations:

- Monitor for worsening signs of redness.

- Educate on limited duration of use.

Administration: Ophthalmic; as directed, usually every 4-6 hours.

OLOPATADINE

Brand Names: Patanol, Pataday

OTC Availability: No

Classification: Antihistamine

Mechanism of Action: Inhibits the release of histamine and other mediators involved in allergic reactions.

Indications:

- Allergic conjunctivitis

Contraindications:

- Hypersensitivity

Side Effects:

- Eye irritation

- Burning or stinging

Nursing Considerations:
- Monitor for worsening signs of allergy.

- Counsel on proper administration technique.

Administration: Ophthalmic; as prescribed, usually twice daily.

OFLOXACIN

Brand Names: Ocuflox

OTC Availability: No

Classification: Fluoroquinolone Antibiotic

Mechanism of Action: Inhibits bacterial DNA gyrase, preventing bacterial DNA replication.

Indications:

- Bacterial conjunctivitis

- Corneal ulcers

Contraindications:

- Hypersensitivity

Side Effects:

- Eye irritation

- Temporary vision changes

Nursing Considerations:

- Monitor for worsening signs of infection.

- Ensure proper administration technique.

Administration: Ophthalmic; as prescribed, often 4-6 times daily.

PILOCARPINE

Brand Names: Isopto Carpine, Pilopine HS

OTC Availability: No

Classification: Miotic Agent

Mechanism of Action: Stimulates the parasympathetic nervous system, resulting in constriction of the pupil and increased outflow of aqueous humor.

Indications:

- Glaucoma

- Ocular surgery

Contraindications:

- Retinal detachment

Side Effects:

- Reduced vision in low light

- Eye irritation

Nursing Considerations:

- Monitor for signs of retinal detachment.

- Assess intraocular pressure regularly.

Administration: Ophthalmic; as prescribed, often 2-4 times daily.

TIMOLOL

Brand Names: Timoptic, Timoptic-XE

OTC Availability: No

Classification: Beta-Blocker

Mechanism of Action: Decreases intraocular pressure by reducing aqueous humor production.

Indications:

- Glaucoma

Contraindications:

- Asthma

- Severe chronic obstructive pulmonary disease (COPD)

Side Effects:

- Burning

- Stinging

Nursing Considerations:

- Monitor intraocular pressure regularly.

- Assess for systemic effects like bradycardia.

Administration: Ophthalmic; as prescribed, usually twice daily.

TOBRAMYCIN

Brand Names: Tobrex

OTC Availability: No

Classification: Aminoglycoside Antibiotic

Mechanism of Action: Inhibits bacterial protein synthesis, resulting in bacterial cell death.

Indications:

- Bacterial conjunctivitis

- Other bacterial eye infections

Contraindications:

- Hypersensitivity

Side Effects:

- Eye irritation

- Stinging

Nursing Considerations:

- Monitor for signs of worsening infection.

- Ensure proper hygiene to avoid cross-contamination.

Administration: Ophthalmic; as prescribed, usually every 4 hours.

TROPICAMIDE

Brand Names: Mydriacyl

OTC Availability: No

Classification: Mydriatic and Cycloplegic Agent

Mechanism of Action: Blocks the action of acetylcholine, causing dilation of the pupil.

Indications:

- Pupil dilation for diagnostic procedures

Contraindications:

- Glaucoma

- Hypersensitivity

Side Effects:
- Temporary blurred vision

- Eye irritation

Nursing Considerations:
- Monitor for signs of glaucoma.

- Warn patient about temporary vision changes.

Administration: Ophthalmic; as prescribed, usually 1-2 drops before exam.

PREDNISOLONE ACETATE

Brand Names: Pred Forte, Omnipred

OTC Availability: No

Classification: Corticosteroid

Mechanism of Action: Suppresses inflammation by inhibiting various components of the inflammatory response.

Indications:

- Eye inflammation

- Post-operative care

Contraindications:

- Viral eye infections

- Fungal eye infections

Side Effects:

- Eye discomfort

- Blurred vision

Nursing Considerations:

- Monitor for signs of infection.

- Educate on proper hygiene to avoid cross-contamination.

Administration: Ophthalmic; as prescribed, usually 2-4 times daily.

Tetrahydrozoline

Brand Names: Visine

OTC Availability: Yes

Classification: Decongestant

Mechanism of Action: Constricts blood vessels in the eyes, reducing redness.

Indications:

- Eye redness

Contraindications:

- Narrow-angle glaucoma

- Hypersensitivity

Side Effects:

- Eye irritation

- Increased intraocular pressure

Nursing Considerations:

- Monitor for worsening signs of redness.

- Educate on limited duration of use.

Administration: Ophthalmic; as directed, usually every 4-6 hours.

PHENYLEPHRINE

Brand Names: Mydfrin, Relief

OTC Availability: No

Classification: Decongestant, Mydriatic Agent

Mechanism of Action: Stimulates alpha-adrenergic receptors, causing pupil dilation and vasoconstriction.

Indications:

- Pupil dilation for diagnostic procedures

- Eye redness

Contraindications:

- Narrow-angle glaucoma

- Hypersensitivity

Side Effects:

- Eye irritation

- Increased intraocular pressure

Nursing Considerations:

- Monitor for signs of glaucoma.

- Warn patient about temporary vision changes.

Administration: Ophthalmic; as prescribed, usually 1-2 drops before exam.

PROPER ADMINISTRATION OF TRANSDERMAL PATCHES

Twelve Rights of Medication Administration

1. **Right Patient**: Confirm the patient's identity using at least two identifiers, like name and date of birth.

2. **Right Medication and Expiration**: Double-check the medication against the prescription. Make sure it has not expired.

3. **Right Dose**: Measure the prescribed dose carefully, using the appropriate instrument.

4. **Right Route**: Confirm that the medication should be given via the intended route (oral, IV, etc.).

5. **Right Time**: Administer the medication at the time prescribed.

6. **Right Documentation**: Record all pertinent information, including medication, dose, time, and any patient reactions.

7. **Right Reason**: Understand the reason for the medication and educate the patient as necessary.

8. **Right to Refuse**: Acknowledge that the patient has the right to refuse medication; their decision should be respected and documented.

9. **Right Response**: Monitor the patient for the expected effects and any possible side effects.

10. **Right Education**: Provide necessary education to the patient or caregiver about the medication.

11. **Right Evaluation**: After administration, evaluate the patient's response to the medication, both therapeutically and for any adverse reactions.

12. **Right to Know**: Ensure the patient and their caregivers understand what medication is being administered, why it is being administered, and what the potential side effects may be.

1. **Preparation:**

   - Verify the prescription, confirming the drug, dose, and frequency according to the "12 Rights of Medication Administration."

- ○ Wash your hands and put on gloves if necessary.

- ○ Prepare the patient by explaining the process and ensuring they're in a comfortable position.

2. **Site Selection:**

- ○ Choose a clean, dry, and hairless area for application.

- ○ The upper arm, chest, or upper back are often recommended sites.

- ○ Avoid areas with cuts, irritation, or excessive movement.

- ○ Rotate sites to avoid skin irritation and enhance absorption.

3. **Patch Preparation:**

- ○ Remove the patch from its packaging.

- ○ If the medication requires it, write the date and time on the patch.

- ○ Do not cut the patch unless specifically directed by a healthcare provider.

4. **Old Patch Removal:**

- ○ If replacing a patch, remove the old one first.

- ○ Fold it in half so the adhesive sides stick together.

- ○ Dispose of it safely, away from children and pets.

5. **Application:**

- Peel the backing off the patch.

- Immediately apply it to the selected site.

- Press down firmly for about 10 seconds to ensure good contact with the skin.

6. Documentation:

- Record the application in the patient's medical record, noting the location, time, and any patient comments.

7. Monitoring:

- Monitor the patient for therapeutic effects and potential side effects.

- Instruct the patient to report any irritation, discomfort, or unusual symptoms.

8. Removal and Disposal:

- Wash hands and put on gloves.

- Carefully peel off the patch.

- Fold it in half so the adhesive sides stick together and dispose of it safely.

BUPRENORPHINE TRANSDERMAL PATCH

Brand Names:

Butrans, Norspan

OTC or Prescription:

Prescription Only

Classification:

Opioid Partial Agonist-Analgesic

Mechanism of Action:

Acts on opioid receptors in the brain and spinal cord to produce analgesia while having a ceiling effect that limits respiratory depression.

Indications:

- Chronic pain management

- Opioid dependence treatment (in some forms)

Contraindications:

- Hypersensitivity to buprenorphine or adhesives

- Severe respiratory insufficiency

- Severe hepatic impairment

Side Effects:

- Nausea

- Constipation

- Headache

- Dizziness

- Drowsiness

Nursing Considerations:

- Monitor for signs of respiratory depression, especially at initiation.

- Assess pain scores regularly to gauge efficacy.

- Watch for signs of opioid withdrawal or overdose.

- Be cautious with other CNS depressants.

Administration:

- **Patch:**

  Colonized

  - Clean and dry the upper arm, upper back, or side of the chest before applying the patch.

- Patches are generally worn for 7 days.

- Do not cut or alter the patch.

- Avoid exposing the patch to heat as it can increase drug absorption.

- Rotate application sites to avoid skin irritation.

- Dispose of properly, fold in half so that the adhesive sides stick together, then dispose of safely.

Fentanyl Transdermal Patch

Brand Names:

Duragesic, Fentanyl Transdermal System

OTC or Prescription:

Prescription Only

Classification:

Opioid Analgesic

Mechanism of Action:

Acts on opioid receptors in the brain and spinal cord to produce analgesia and sedation.

Indications:

Management of chronic pain in patients who require continuous opioid analgesia for an extended period.

Contraindications:

- Hypersensitivity to Colonized Opioid-naive patients

- Acute or postoperative pain

- Respiratory depression

- Paralytic ileus

Side Effects:
- Respiratory depression

- Constipation

- Nausea

- Drowsiness

- Confusion

Nursing Considerations:
- Use extreme caution in dose calculation; fentanyl is highly potent.

- Monitor respiratory rate, blood pressure, and pain relief regularly.

- Use caution with other CNS depressants or alcohol.

- Be aware of signs of fentanyl overdose, including slowed breathing, extreme sleepiness, and difficulty walking or talking.

Administration:
- **Patch:**

  - Applied to a clean, dry, hairless area of the skin on the upper arm, chest, or back.

  - The patch is usually changed every 72 hours.

- Do not use heat sources like heating pads or hot water baths on the patch as it may increase drug absorption.

- Rotate application sites to avoid skin irritation.

- Fold the used patch in half, sticky side in, and dispose of it safely away from children and pets.

Nitroglycerin Transdermal Patch

Brand Names:

Nitro-Dur, Minitran, Transderm-Nitro

OTC or Prescription:

Prescription Only

Classification:

Anti-Anginal, Vasodilator

Mechanism of Action:

Releases nitric oxide, which relaxes smooth muscles in the blood vessels, leading to dilation. This reduces the workload on the heart and relieves angina.

Indications:

- Prevention of angina pectoris

- Treatment of chronic angina

Contraindications:

- Hypersensitivity to nitroglycerin or other nitrates

- Severe anemia

- Recent myocardial infarction

- Hypotension

Side Effects:
- Headache

- Dizziness

- Flushing

- Hypotension

Nursing Considerations:
- Monitor blood pressure and heart rate.

- Rotate patch sites to prevent skin irritation.

- Instruct the patient to report severe headaches or persistent chest pain.

- Patients should sit or lie down when applying the patch to avoid dizziness or falls.

Administration:
- **Patch**:

  - Apply to a clean, hairless area on the chest or upper arm.

  - Remove old patch before applying a new one.

  - Typical use involves a 12- to 14-hour "on" period followed by a nitrate-free interval to reduce tolerance.

- Do not cut the patch.

Scopolamine Transdermal Patch

Brand Names:

Transderm Scop

OTC or Prescription:

Prescription Only

Classification:

Anticholinergic, Antiemetic

Mechanism of Action:

Inhibits the action of acetylcholine at muscarinic receptors in the vestibular system, thereby preventing nausea and vomiting.

Indications:

- Motion sickness prevention

- Postoperative nausea and vomiting

Contraindications:

- Hypersensitivity to scopolamine or other belladonna alkaloids

- Angle-closure glaucoma

- Severe hepatic or renal impairment

Side Effects:

- Dry mouth

- Dizziness

- Blurred vision

- Drowsiness

Nursing Considerations:

- Monitor for anticholinergic side effects like dry mouth, urinary retention, and constipation.

- Monitor for signs of delirium or confusion in elderly patients.

- Remove patch immediately if hallucinations or severe confusion occur.

Administration:

- **Patch:**

  - Apply to a clean, dry, and hairless area behind the ear.

  - Typically worn for up to 3 days.

  - Do not cut or alter the patch.

  - Remove the old patch before applying a new one.

  - Wash hands thoroughly after handling to avoid accidental transfer to eyes or mouth.

RESOURCES AND BOOK RECOMMENDATIONS

1. **Davis's Drug Guide for Nurses**

2. **Mosby's Nursing Drug Reference**

3. **Nursing2023 Drug Handbook (Nursing Drug Handbook)**

Drug Guides:

1. **Davis's Drug Guide for Nurses** - Comprehensive, up-to-date drug guide for nurses.

2. **Mosby's Nursing Drug Reference** - Offers a user-friendly guide to over 1,000 drugs.

3. **Nursing2023 Drug Handbook (Nursing Drug Handbook)** - Provides quick access to current, accurate informa-

tion on over 3,000 brand-name and generic drugs.

4. **Saunders Nursing Drug Handbook** - Includes the most recent FDA-approved drugs and is well organized.

General Nursing References:

1. **Fundamentals of Nursing** by Patricia A. Potter - Covers basic nursing concepts, theories, and practices.

2. **Medical-Surgical Nursing: Concepts for Interprofessional Collaborative Care** - Focuses on adult health conditions with a medical-surgical focus.

3. **Lippincott Manual of Nursing Practice** - Comprehensive nursing manual covering a wide array of topics.

Specialized Areas:

1. **Critical Care Nursing: Diagnosis and Management** - A detailed book focusing on critical care nursing.

2. **Pediatric Nursing: The Critical Components of Nursing Care** - For those interested in pediatric nursing.

3. **Psychiatric Nursing: Contemporary Practice** - Covers the psychiatric nursing landscape.

Online Resources:

1. **UpToDate** - Comprehensive evidence-based clinical resource.

2. **Medscape** - Includes news, drug information, and journals in the field of healthcare.

3. **The Cochrane Library** - Collection of databases containing high-quality, independent evidence for healthcare decision-making.

Journals:

1. **Journal of Advanced Nursing**

2. **Nursing Outlook**

3. **American Journal of Nursing (AJN)**

These resources are often recommended for healthcare professionals, including nurses, to keep up-to-date with the latest clinical guidelines, medications, and treatment procedures.